Essential Oils and Aromatherapy

A Beginner's Guide to Making and Using Essential Oils at Home for Skincare and Beauty Products

Josephine Simon

DISCLAIMER AND COPYRIGHT

CONTENTS

INTRODUCTION

Most of us are aware about Aromatherapy oils and their basic benefits. Almost every other person craves for an aromatherapy oil massage or invests in aromatherapy hair, skin, and beauty products. This miracle product is your one-stop solution for most of your beauty concerns.

Whether you have patchy, dry, wrinkled, or tanned skin, and/or dull hair, essential oils can help address all these problems in a safe manner. Essential oils do not cost much and can be considered as one of the most affordable ways to maintain healthy skin in a natural manner. We often end up spending a fortune over various skin and hair products that may or may not show results.

With aromatherapy oils, you will definitely start seeing results after regular application, although you need to remember that nothing happens overnight. This is only possible with regular usage over a period of time.

You may think that aromatherapy oils are merely a fad that has been advocated by the skincare and beauty industry, but the outcomes of using these oils may pleasantly surprise you. That being said, we wish to strongly recommend consulting a medical practitioner about the amount of its usage.

This eBook also contains different recipes to make your own skin and hair products using essential oils. These products can be stored in the refrigerator for months without their quality getting deteriorated.

Through this eBook, we want to educate our readers about using aromatherapy oils to, to reap you the maximum benefits. We hope you enjoy reading the eBook and make aromatherapy oils an essential part of skin and hair care routine.

WHAT IS AROMATHERAPY?

Aromatherapy is both an art and a science. The essential oils of Aromatherapy have been used since ancient civilizations, the first documented usage being by the Egyptians around 3000 BC. In those days, it was used as incense for worship. Now it's used for its numerous health and beauty benefits.

Today, aromatherapy has developed and taken up many forms and applications. It is often accompanied by the use of essential oils. These oils are easily absorbed by the body and help in treating many different types of ailments.

After absorption, they travel through the bloodstream and cover different parts of the body. Thus, on application, they offer you a sense of relief, and you can experience your body de-stressing. This approach to treatment does not only address the symptoms but also aims to solve the underlying problems that have caused the symptoms.

Benefits of Aromatherapy

There are many reasons why Aromatherapy has been accepted as a popular treatment by people around the globe. Most important is aromatherapy's ability to treat the patient in a holistic manner. Factors like medical background of the patient along with her lifestyle, diet, and behavioral patterns are taken into consideration, well in advance of the commencement of the treatment.

This is why a lot of research that has been conducted on aromatherapy and its benefits have found some interesting results:

- Usage of aromatherapy over a long period of time has shown to strengthen the immune system.
- It helps fight against infections and illnesses.
- Aromatherapy is a guaranteed stress reliever. It means that all stress-related ailments like constipation, headaches, joint pain, and so on can be treated via aromatherapy.
- Aromatherapy does not base its efficacy on animal testing, as it has been, over the centuries, tried on humans and proven to have no side-effects.

What are essential oils?

Almost each part of a plant has oils stored inside it. The extraction of these essential oils forms the basis of all aromatherapy-based treatments. Other than their name, essential oils share no other common characteristic with the oils we encounter in our daily lives. They are neither sticky nor are they colored, unless they are some of the heavier essential oils. Essential oils contain the very essence of the plant from which they are extracted. Due to their intensity, a drop or two works magic and is usually more than enough.

Many people confuse essential oils with perfumes or fragrances. Essential oils might have a fragrance of their own, but they are in no way similar to the latter two. Unlike essential oils, perfumes are artificially extracted or sometimes created with the addition of external and artificial substances. Therefore, other than their smell, they offer nothing else, unlike essential oils, which are replete with therapeutic benefits.

Carrier oils are another important aspect that you need to understand to fully comprehend the application of essential oils. An essential oil is always accompanied by a carrier oil, like grape-seed oil for example, as they help dilute the essential oil. This blend is then used for application on the skin and the mixture is easily absorbed.

How does aromatherapy work?

Some studies have shown that the smells generated by essential oils stimulate the part of the brain that is in charge of olfactory functions. After this, the brain releases chemicals that in turn relieve stress and cause the body to calm down.

Aromatherapy and beauty

The beauty industry has witnessed a revolution in the recent past. While the good news is that it has evolved to newer and more progressive avenues of cosmetic enhancement, the bad news is that it has also brought with it increasing pressure to undergo painful, irreversible, and dangerous procedures, so as to live up to a finer image of beauty.

Aromatherapy has acted as an elixir in these times of dramatic artificiality. It has helped users regain a pure and organic beauty that can only come from a closer connection to nature and its extractions.

There are many reasons why aromatherapy is preferred over other cosmetic and beauty procedures.

Some of them are mentioned here:

- It is completely safe without any side effects. It causes no harm to the body in any way.
- Its effects are long lasting, and continued usage over the years has shown that it can drastically improve and treat beauty related problems.
- Its effects are proven to be beneficial for hair growth. It improves hair quality and can address problems like split ends and easy breakability.
- Possibly the most attractive quality about aromatherapy is that its usage has shown to fight different signs of aging. Its application as an anti-aging treatment has made it hugely popular with women all over the world, be they actors, celebrities, or housewives.

DIFFERENT TYPES OF ESSENTIAL OILS

Essential Oils have gained in popularity over the past few years. Over time, people have started to realize that essential oils and Aromatherapy can benefit their skin and hair immensely. Therefore, rather than spending a fortune on a truck load of cosmetic products, people are finding it easier to maintain their beauty using these multipurpose essential oils.

There are numerous types of oils that can offer youthful-looking skin and hair, and also go a long way in helping you stay fit. These oils have antibacterial, anti-fungal, or anti-inflammatory properties that can prevent different allergies and inflammation. There are almost about 90 essential oil varieties, found all around the world, which are used for different purposes in different cultures.

Although the usage of essential oils is an extremely safe way of treating or maintaining your beauty, if taken in excess, it can cause certain side effects. Try not to go on a rampage and use any random essential oil that you get your hands on. **If you have no knowledge about what it consists of and how it**

works, it is important that you consult a medical professional before you go ahead and use it. A medical practitioner will be able to tell you the exact amount of usage and its properties.

Below, you will find a list of ten of the most used essentials oils and their properties.

Peppermint

Peppermint can instantly refresh you and make you feel active. It helps in treating nausea, bad breath, and many other problems. Peppermint oil can be used to treat stomach problems (caused due to inflammation), applied on itchy skin or be used merely to feel fresh throughout the day.

A few drops of peppermint oil in your bath water can shield you against congestion problems or soothe inflamed parts of your body. Not just that, peppermint is one of the key ingredients used in making oils that can help you alleviate PMS pain. Just gently massage it on the lower part of your stomach and leave it overnight. It will offer immense relief from excruciating PMS pain.

Additionally, it is used to treat common colds, migraines, and even used to enhance your concentration. People with focus issues also can benefit from regular usage of essential oils like peppermint.

Lavender

A lot of medical practitioners swear by lavender oils and its benefits. These oils have an extremely gentle fragrance and are highly effective in curing a lot of skin problems. Whether it is sunburned skin, acne, or pimples, it works wonders.

It is also used for massaging hair. Regular usage of this oil will not only make your hair healthier, but it can also save it from breakage. It has antibacterial properties that can help fight bacteria from your body. Like peppermint oil, lavender oils also help to cure digestion problems.

Sesame

Sesame oil may not smell that great, but its benefits are definitely worth it. It has high skin moisturizing characteristics that will ensure your skin remains hydrated and moist all the time.

This oil works wonders for people who have dry skin issues and want dewy, glowing skin. You don't have to undergo numerous beauty treatments and facials, which can drill a hole into your pockets. It also has SPF, which will prevent your skin from getting burned due to excess exposure the sun.

Rose

Rose oil has a reputation of being a "woman-friendly" oil. It smells just like a fresh rose and can lighten up your mood within a few minutes. Rose oils can also be used instead of a body spray.

This mildly distilled oil is a top favorite essential oil among aromatherapists. It is also known as the "the perfect oil for a woman." This is due to the fact that it is known to balance out a woman's hormones during her menopausal stage. It can instantly bring you PMS relief.

Geranium

Geranium oil has astringent properties that help in refreshing skin. Its styptic aspects calm inflammations and stop hemorrhaging. It also helps provide relief from PMS symptoms.

It can be used to treat acne and oily skin. It increases circulation and decreases bloating. The oil can reduce the appearance of scars and marks and is helpful to get rid of body odor.

Apart from that, it can be utilized to contract blood vessels for reducing the fine lines and wrinkles on your face. In other terms, it acts as antiaging oil.

Pine

Its antiseptic, antibacterial, and analgesic properties make it a favorite with holistic health experts. Pine oil is said to help treat skin issues including psoriasis, eczema, and pimples. It speeds up metabolism, acts as an antidote to food poisoning, helps ease joint pain and arthritis, kill germs, and battles respiratory problems that come along with cough and cold.

Clove

This is a popular choice for dental issues, including tooth and gum pain. Some people even recommend using it for bad breath. Clove oil is antiseptic, so diluted versions can treat bug bites, cuts, and scrapes. The other uses include soothing earaches, use in solving digestive problems, clearing nasal congestion, and alleviating stomachaches and headaches. Spicy clove oil is one of the main ingredients in a lot of balms as well.

Black Pepper

Though it may not be as sweet-smelling as the other floral entries on this list, black pepper oil holds on its own as an essential oil in our natural health armory. Pepper is one of the world's most valuable spices because of its healing properties, which include aiding digestion, soothing cramps and convulsions, warming muscles to ease joint pain and arthritis, and curing bacterial infections.

Lemon Balm

Lemon balm essential oil, also known as *Melissa officinalis* is a miracle product. It acts as an antibiotic, soothes your body, alleviates pain, calms you down, and prevents inflammation and ulcers.

Essential oils may be a little more expensive than other oils such as coconut oil or hair care oils. However, when you use these oils, you will realize that they are worth the price. Influences contributing towards its price include the botanical factors, the origin of the oils, the quality of the distillery, and quantity of oil produced.

Essential oils can be bought as blends of several essential oils. These mixtures of oils can solve your issues of buying individual oils, thereby saving a lot of your hard-earned money.

APPLICATIONS OF ESSENTIAL OILS

When it comes to skincare, we somehow tend to blindly believe any claim that different beauty products make. We don't even think twice before using the creams that are prescribed to us by our dermatologists in hopes of enhancing our beauty with better skin. We fail to understand that though these creams may provide us with short-term benefits, they also contain chemicals, which can, in the long run, seriously harm our skin.

How much better is it to go a natural way, i.e. the way of aromatherapy and application of essential oils to better our skin without sustaining any long term damages? This way we'll not only achieve a flawless skin in the most natural way with the least use of chemicals, but also gain benefits like reduced stress due to aromatherapy that OTC creams would never be able to achieve.

Aromatherapy is a method whereby we use plant components, i.e. the essential oils that we get from different plants, and combine them with different aromas for the betterment of our skin. Aromatherapy allows the oils to be absorbed by our bloodstream to give us long term effects for our health.

Aromatherapy for skin is a form of medicine that has been in practice for a very long time. It is extremely beneficial in curing skin diseases, soothing dry or injured skin, helping in prevention of aging, curing pimples and black heads, and much more.

Before using any of these oils on your skin, you must know your skin type and what you are allergic to. It is essential you choose the oils with extreme care. Before putting the oil anywhere near your face, it is important that you first conduct a small patch test on your wrist to know if you are allergic to that oil or not.

These oils can be used either in combinations of two or more or individually according to your skin type. Ideally, you should add 2 drops of this oil to 3.4 oz. (100 ml) of your everyday cleanser or moisturizer.

Mentioned below are some aromatherapy essential oils and their application for various skin types, skincare uses, and beautification purpose:

- **General skin**
  Sandalwood, lavender, and rose

- **Dry Skin**

  Cedarwood, clary sage, carrot seed, geranium, lavender, jasmine, orange, rose, Roman chamomile, palmarosa, rosewood, mandarin-petitgrain, sandalwood, hydrosol, carrot seed, lavender, rose, ylang-ylang

- **For combination skin**

  Lavender, geranium, rosewood, rose hydrosol, neroli hydrosol, ylang-ylang

- **Cracked Skin**

  Patchouli, sandalwood, cajeput, Roman & German chamomile, vetiver lavender, Benzoin

- **Oily Skin**

  Roman & German chamomile, geranium, lavender, ylang-ylang, lemon, peppermint, Cedarwood, cypress, calendula infusion, patchouli, sandalwood, frankincense, juniper, yarrow, coriander, clary, Melissa, lime distilled, thyme linalool, spike lavender, rose, grapefruit

- **Sensitive Skin**

  Roman & German chamomile, palmarosa, neroli, Rose, rosewood, carrot, angelica, chamomile or yarrow hydrosols, jasmine

- **Acne**

  Lavender, tea tree, rose geranium, sandalwood, mints, basil, German chamomile, palmarosa, grapefruit, manuka, atlas Cedarwood, yarrow hydrosol, cajeput

- **Black heads**

  Peppermints, lemongrass, coriander, thymus vulgaris

- **Hydrating**

  Sweet orange, tangerine, most hydrosols, neroli, palmarosa, mandarin

- **Infections**

  German chamomile, eucalyptus, myrtle, lavender, manuka, , thyme linalool, myrrh, Roman chamomile, rosemary, spikenard, tea tree, calendula, palmarosa, niaouli, laurel, rosewood

- **Inflammation**

  Helichrysum, carrot seed, galbanum German & Roman chamomiles, clary, myrtle, rosewood, myrrh, angelica, yarrow, witch hazel or chamomile hydrosols

- **Mature, aged skin, wrinkles**

  Frankincense, galbanum, geranium, Carrot seed, elemi, Cistus, myrrh, rose, Clary, rosewood, sages, cypress, fennel, lavender, neroli, patchouli, fennel, Sea Buckthorn Berry Extract, Rose Hip Extract

- **Itching**

  Jasmine, lavender, peppermint, helichrysum, Roman chamomile

BENEFITS OF ESSENTIAL OILS FOR SKINCARE

Since time immemorial, beauty has been enhanced through the use of natural ingredients. From Cleopatra bathing in milk to Indian goddesses dousing themselves in turmeric and sandalwood-infused concoctions, nature has proved to be a treasure trove of skin elixirs. Not only do essential oils work wonders in reversing adverse skin conditions but also help in keeping skin looking young and beautiful while staying healthy.

They make for great alternatives to commercial cosmetic products, as the risk of side effects that harsh chemicals can cause is greatly reduced. They can also be much more effective in terms of results.

Here is a comprehensive look at the various skincare benefits of essential oils:-

Moisturizing

All skin types, regardless of being normal, dry, or oily need good amounts of moisturizing to keep them healthy and supple. Essential oils are one of the most widely used products to help serve the purpose of skin moisturizing. Sandalwood and rose are the two most preferred oils, mainly for their therapeutic fragrances. Despite lacking a pleasant smell, coconut oil is also extremely useful in moisturizing skin and can effectively fight off weather-related skin dryness. Lanolin oil is also very effective in keeping the skin moist for long periods of time.

Anti-viral

Bergamot oil possesses anti-viral properties and can be used to treat herpes and viral skin rashes. Tea-tree oil also possesses anti-viral properties and can be used to provide relief from shingles.

Anti-fungal

Oils such as cinnamon, clove, coriander, and lavender have anti-fungal properties and can be used to effectively curtail athlete's foot and scalp-related fungal infections. They also help in reducing the inflammation, itching, and redness whilst providing a cooling and soothing effect on the skin.

Anti-bacterial

Neem oil is known to possess anti-bacterial properties and is widely used in the treatment of Acne Vulgaris. Teenagers are at most risk of developing acne, Dabbing a little oil on the affected area will help in drying out the inflammations and effectively reducing the itching and redness.

Astringent properties

Lemon oil, orange oil, and other citrus-based oils are known to fight off and keep skin oil at bay. They help in closing up the pores that are responsible in releasing sebum. It is therefore a good idea to scrub the face and apply lemon or rosemary oil to close the pores. Reduced sizes of pores aid in making skin aesthetically pleasing.

Cell growth

Rosehip oil is a good skin elixir because it contains Omega 3, 6, and 9, vitamin C, lycopene, and linoleic acids, which help in healthy cell generation. This in turn helps in boosting collagen, which causes skin to regain vital, vigor, and elasticity. Geranium oil is also extremely effective in helping the face generate healthy skin cells. Lemon oil is anti-carcinogenic and can be used to fight cancerous skin cells.

Odor control

People suffering from body odor can employ jasmine and geranium oils to combat and control the condition effectively. Geranium oil helps in curbing the bacteria responsible for causing body odor. The fragrance of jasmine oil helps in promoting a pleasant body odor.

Youth restoration

Sandalwood oil is extremely effective in reducing fine lines and wrinkles. Applying a thin layer of this oil on the face before retiring to bed can help in restoring youthful skin. Rosehip oil helps in adding back skin firmness which can help in lifting up sagging skin.

Promote fairness

Lemon oil is known to lighten a person's skin tone. Dabbing on a little oil over dark skin everyday can help in lightening the complexion. Sesame and jojoba oil can also be used for the same purpose. Bergamot oil is extremely effective in evening out skin tone and can be used in dealing with patchy skin color.

Scar treatment

Geranium oil as well as lemon oil is very effective in reducing scars. Acne scars, post-operative stretch marks, pregnancy-related stretch marks, and wound scars can all be reduced using geranium or lemon oil. Bergamot can be used in treating cracked heels.

Sensitive skin

People with sensitive skin who cannot use commercial products to cleanse and moisturize face out of fear of breaking out into rashes can safely use chamomile oil to effectively and naturally clean and moisturize their skin.

Men's skin

Men's skin is a bit harsher and coarser than women's. Oils such as patchouli, bay, ginger, and cypress can be employed to tackle men's skin needs. Patchouli is used to balance skin oil and keep acne at bay. It is also used in curing athlete's foot. Bay and cypress are also used to treat oily acne-prone skin. Chamomile oil is effective in keeping men's skin soft.

Baby's skin

Babies have very sensitive skins, and using commercial cosmetic products containing chemicals can be risky. Essential oils make for great alternative choices. Jojoba oil can be safely used to massage baby skin. The oil helps to seal in moisture and relieve dry skin and also helps in the treatment of diaper rashes.

Insect bites

Certain insect bites cause pain accompanied by stinging sensations. Applying chemical-laden commercial products can simply worsen the case. Essential oils such as peppermint, thyme, and eucalyptus can be used to provide relief from tick, mosquito, and flea bites. These oils will not only help with the pain and itching but also do not allow any skin scars to remain. Eucalyptus oil can also be applied as a preventive measure when heading out into the wilderness or other insect-infested areas.

Glowing skin

Almond oil can be used to lend the face a healthy glow. The oil helps in causing dull lifeless skin develop a healthy sheen while also preventing it from going dry. Olive oil can also be employed to make the face develop a healthy glow.

MAKING ESSENTIAL OILS AT HOME: INGREDIENTS AND APPARATUS

Although it is easy to buy essential oils from your local drug or grocery stores, they can be a bit on the expensive side. You can instead make these oils at home by extracting them directly from raw materials such as herbs, flowers, and fruit peels.

Depending on the degree of concentration and purity, three types of methods to extract essential oils can be used. The most widely used method is known as the distillation method, in which a special oil extraction device called a distiller is used. This particular method is most preferred as it gives off the strongest and most concentrated of results.

Carrier oil and infusion are the other two types of oil extraction methods.

Let us look at each one in detail.

Distillation Method

The distiller or still, is an apparatus that is used to extract oils from herbs, flowers, and fruits. The basic mechanism that a distiller employs to extract the oil involves the heating and cooling down of the raw materials in close successions and ultimately collecting the oil.

A distiller has three components – a heating device, a steam carrier tube, and a collector. The heater is a vessel that helps in heating up the raw materials in boiling water to allow them to release their oil. The heat then escapes in the form of steam along with the essential oil.

The steam-containing oil is then passed through copper tubing that is immersed in ice cold water. The cold water helps in condensing the steam and turning it into liquid, with the oil still intact. The water is then collected and further allowed to cool. After it cools completely, the oil collects at the top and can be easily skimmed off.

Distillers are available in most hardware stores and can also be bought online. A standard oil distiller can cost anywhere between a few hundred to several hundred dollars depending on quality and size.

As expensive as it might sound, a distiller is a great investment as it can be used to extract any amount of essential oils from any number of raw materials, making it cost effective in the long run. But if price is a factor, then a distiller can easily be made at home.

The quality of oil output might differ and not be as high as store-bought oils, but homemade distillers can help in extracting good quality essential oils. The process of building a distiller might be simple, but you will be required to conduct several trial and error methods to arrive at the right way of extracting the best concentration and quality of oil.

Building a distiller

A distiller can easily be built at home with raw materials purchased online or from hardware stores. If it is difficult to find a pressure cooker then it can be substituted with a tea kettle.

Here are the raw materials needed to build a distiller:

1. Standard Pressure cooker – 1
2. 10 mm Copper wire – 10 meters
3. Plastic tube – 2 inches
4. Large plastic tub – 1
5. Large glass jar – 1

Method:

- Prepare the lid of the pressure cooker by blocking all other valves and keeping only the steam valve open.
- Bend the copper wire in such a way that it coils one fold in the middle. You can either do it yourself by wrapping it around a mini cylinder or have a metal worker do it for you.
- Place the rubber tube over the steam valve so that it fits perfectly and no steam can escape. You can also further secure it using a water proof sealant.

Your distiller is now ready. The correct method of using the distiller to extract oil is as follows:

- Place the cooker on top of the gas stove.
- Collect a substantial amount of your raw materials (orange peels, lavender flowers, and more) and place them inside the cooker so that only an inch of space remains at the top.
- Pour water from a recently boiled kettle over the raw materials, making sure to use three parts water to one part material.
- Close the lid of the cooker tightly, and turn on the gas.

- Place a large tub of cold water next to the cooker and immerse as much of the copper tube in it as possible.
- Place the open end of the copper tube inside a glass jar which will act as the receiver of the oil-containing water.
- Once the jar fills up or you have collected a satisfactory amount of oil, switch off the gas, and allow the collected water to cool down.
- After it cools, the essential oil will float at the top and can be easily skimmed and collected.
- Place the oil in a small glass bottle marked with the name of the oil.

Your essential oil is now ready to use.

Note: The collected oil might be extremely concentrated and should be diluted using carrier oils such as coconut or olive oil before being applied onto skin. The ratio of carrier to essential oil will depend on the concentration level of the latter.

Carrier oil method

Essential oils can also be extracted without the help of a distiller. The results might not be the same, but it is an easier and cheaper method of extracting the oil.

No special apparatus will be required for this process, and only a few household items will be needed.

The following things are required for the carrier oil method of extraction

1. Large utensil for boiling – 1
2. Rose petals or any other raw materials – 1 cup
3. Carrier oils (coconut, almond) – ½ cup
4. Vitamin E oil – 2 drops
5. Fine cloth strainer – 1
6. Dark glass bottles for storage

Method:

- Place the flowers or fruit peels inside the utensil along with the carrier oil.
- Add in the vitamin E oil, and give it a good mix.
- Place on low heat for four hours.

- Do not bring the mixture to a boil, and maintain a gentle heat supply.
- Switch off the heat, and let the mixture cool down before passing it through a fine cloth sieve.
- Collect it in glass jars and allow it to mature for a couple of days.

The essential oil collected through this method is generally less concentrated as compared to the oils made through the distilled method and can be used as is for cosmetic purposes.

Infusion method

The infusion method is an even simpler method that can be employed to make essential oils at home. The resultant oil will probably be the least concentrated but will still serve as a great alternative to expensive store bought oils.

Infusion method will require the following materials:

1. Carrier oil (coconut, sunflower, olive) – ½ cup
2. Oil raw materials (Flower petals, fruit peels, herbs) – 1 cup
3. Glass jar – 1

Method:

- Place the carrier oil along with the raw materials in an air tight glass jar and give it a good mix.
- Close the lid tightly and place the jar in a dark room.
- Let the oil infuse with the raw materials for a minimum of two weeks.
- Strain the mixture and collect it in a second jar.

The oil is ready to be used.

Regardless of which method is employed to make the essential oils, they will always be better options than store bought products as they will be free from any form of chemicals. Also, the costs to make them will work out to be much less than the cost of commercial oils.

Important safety measures

- Be sure to use only glass bottles for storing the essential oils as any other materials such as plastic can react with the oils and modify their composition.

- Always mark your oils with their date of creation. Essential oils come with shelf lives and will not be safe to be used after their expiration dates.

- Store them in dark rooms away from direct sunlight so that their potency and shelf life can increase. Using dark color glass bottle also helps.

- Cleanse the distiller thoroughly after every use and discard any residual fragrance and oil from previous processes as to not interfere with subsequent usage.

RECIPES FOR SKINCARE PRODUCTS USING ESSENTIALS OILS

Commercial cosmetics these days are laden with dangerous chemicals that might be causing more harm to the skin than good. From fairness creams to perfumes, almost all cosmetics have a rather questionable ingredient list, which will make you think twice before using it on your body.

Further worsening the cause is the testing of the product on animals. Cosmetic companies often subject animals to harsh chemical experiments, capable of disfiguring their bodies and even causing their deaths.

However, that does not mean we stop taking baths or applying creams. Our bodies will need a little nourishment to maintain a healthy skin and shiny hair.

Homemade products, therefore, are a great alternative to store-bought ones. They can easily be made at home and you need not worry about any harsh chemicals entering our bodies can be eliminated.

Body Butter

Body butters are thick body lotions that are great for relieving dry skin. Applying just a little every day can help prevent the skin from drying out and help maintain a youthful glow.

Strawberry body butter recipe

Ingredients:
- Shea butter – 1 ¾ oz. (50 grams)
- Coconut oil – 1 oz. (30 grams)
- Strawberry essential oil – 15 drops
- Edible red food color – 1 teaspoon

Method:
- In a double boiler, place the coconut oil and the Shea butter, and melt until it softens up and reaches a creamy texture.
- Add in the essential oil along with the food coloring.
- Give it a good mix and allow it to cool down.

- Transfer the mix into a glass bowl. Using an electric hand blender, whip the mixture for 2-4 minutes. (The whipping adds in air into the mix and makes it light and fluffy.)

The butter can be stored in food grade plastic containers that are generally available in dollar stores.

The shelf life of the butter will match the shelf life of the coconut oil, so make sure to mark the butter with its expiration date.

Basil body butter recipe

Basil is an herb that is known to regenerate healthy skin cells thereby helping to keep skin firm and reduce wrinkles. The butter also aids in reducing scar marks and dryness.

Ingredients:

- Shea Butter – 1 ¾ oz. (50 grams)
- Jojoba oil – 1 teaspoon
- Coconut oil – 1 oz. (30 grams)
- Vitamin E oil – 1 teaspoon
- Basil essential oil – 10 to15 drops

Method:

- Place the Shea butter and coconut oil in a double boiler, and melt until it reaches a creamy consistency.
- Add the jojoba and Vitamin E oil along with 15 drops of the basil essential oil.
- Give it all a good mix and allow it to cool down.
- Use an electric blender to whip the mixture for 2-4 minutes.
- Transfer into a glass or food grade plastic bottle.

The butter will stay good for around a month.

Body Scrubs

Body scrubs make for great skin exfoliators and assist in getting rid of dry, dead skin. Lemon acts in two ways by aiding in removing excessive oil and also in closing up oil pores thanks to its astringent properties.

Lemon sugar body scrub

Ingredients:
- Refined Demerara sugar (granulated brown sugar) – ½ cup
- Coconut oil – 2 tablespoons
- Lemon essential oil – 5 drops

Method:
- Mix the sugar and coconut oil together such that the oil coats all of the sugar granules.
- Add in the lemon oil and give it a good mix.
- Store in glass canisters for easy access

The amount of lemon oil to be used will depend on how strong an astringent you would want to make of it.

Moisturizing Body Scrub

Ingredients:

- Shea Butter – ½ cup
- Coarse Sea Salt – ½ cup
- Olive Oil – 2 tablespoons
- Vanilla essential oil – 10 to 12 drops

Method:

- Place the Shea butter on a double boiler and soften it.
- Add in the olive and vanilla essential oil and give it a good mix.
- Place the coarse salt in the jar that will house the scrub.
- Pour the Shea Butter mixture over the salt and give it a good mix.

The scrub will act as an exfoliator whilst also supplying the skin with moisture.

Sunscreens

Sunscreens are lotions that protect the skin from absorbing the harmful UVA and UVB rays of the sun. Applying sunscreen before stepping out into the sun should be a routine habit regardless of the weather.

Raspberry, Carrot Essential Oil Sunscreen

Ingredients:
- Coconut oil – ½ cup
- Almond oil – ½ cup
- Shea Butter – ¼ cup
- Raspberry seed essential oil – 15 drops
- Carrot seed oil – 15 drops
- Raspberry essence (optional) – 5 drops

Method:
- Place the coconut oil, almond oil, and Shea butter in a measuring jar or a steel utensil and place over a double boiler.
- Let the mixture melt. Turn off the heat when it reaches a creamy texture.
- Add the raspberry and carrot seed oil along with the raspberry essence.

- Give the mixture a good stir and transfer into a food grade plastic jar or a glass jar. Let it cool completely.

Apply half an hour before stepping out into the sun. The sunscreen provides for a total SPF of 20-25 depending on the quantity of the ingredients used. Reapply sunscreen every 4 hours.

Do not add any citrus essential oils as they can increase skin sensitivity towards sun rays.

Note: An additional ingredient called "zinc oxide" may be used to make the sunscreen a little stronger. The ingredient can be bought from a pharmacy or from online sites such as Amazon. Make sure that you buy "non-nano" zinc oxide. Be very careful in handling the zinc oxide, making sure no amount of it is inhaled.

Face Masks

Face masks make for great skin rejuvenators. Not only do they help in closing the open pores, they also lend the skin a healthy glow.

Face mask for oily skin

Ingredients:
- Fuller's Earth – ½ cup
- Clove oil – 15 drops
- Cinnamon bark oil – 5 drops

Method:
- Mix all the ingredients together and store in an airtight container.

How to use:
- Take a coin-sized amount of the mixture, and add in a little water to make a thick paste.
- Apply evenly all over the skin, concentrating on the pimple-prone areas.
- Allow it to stay for 15 minutes or until it completely dries up.
- Wash off with cold water.

Clove essential oil is an excellent anti-acne ingredient and Fuller's Earth helps a lot in closing up pores.

Skin Whitening Mask

Ingredients:

- Milk powder – ½ cup
- Powdered oatmeal – ¼ cup
- Rose essential oil – 5 drops
- Sandalwood oil – 10 drops
- Rose essence – 2 drops

Method:

- Combine the milk powder along with the rose and sandalwood oils, and give it a good mix.
- Add in the essence and transfer into a plastic jar.

How to use:

- Take a coin-sized amount of the mix and add a few drops of rose water to make a thick paste.
- Apply evenly all over the face and wash off after 20 minutes.
- Repeat the process twice a week.

Lip Balms

Approaching winters are not just a cause of worry for the characters of the Game of Thrones but also for our poor lips. Chapped lips can be painful and unsightly. Lip balms can provide with great relief. They don't just help with the chaffing but also provide moisture.

Carrot seed oil lip balm

Ingredients:

- Carrot seed oil – 2 tablespoons
- Vitamin E oil – ¼ tablespoon
- Shea butter – 2 tablespoons

Method:

- Slightly warm all the ingredients in a double boiler.
- Allow it to cool before transferring it into a small glass or plastic bottle.
- A few drops of lavender essential oil maybe added to enhance the flavor of the lip balm.

Chocolate lip balm

Ingredients:-

- Coconut oil – 2 tablespoons
- Vitamin E oil – ¼ teaspoon
- Shea butter – 2 tablespoons
- Good quality cocoa powder – 1 tablespoon

Method:

- Lightly melt the Shea butter along with the vitamin E and coconut oil on a double boiler.
- Remove from heat and add the cocoa powder and give it a good mix.
- Enjoy your chocolate lip balm.

Note: Do not lick lips after applying the lip balm as the Shea butter can cause dryness inside the mouth.

Hair Care

Hair oils and serums are a great way to keep hair healthy as not only do they help in strengthening the hair roots, but they also add shine to the hair.

Multi-purpose hair oil

Ingredients:
- Coconut oil – ¼ cup, melted
- Jojoba oil – 5 tablespoons
- Basil essential oil – 2 tablespoons
- Tea tree oil – 2 tablespoons

Method:
- Pour all the oils in a jar and give it a good shake.
- Apply the oil an hour before washing off with the homemade lavender essential oil shampoo.
- Massage the oil into the scalp using circular motions.

The basil oil helps in curbing dandruff and also provides relief from dull, dry hair. The coconut and jojoba oils help in adding moisture to the hair and also a healthy shine.

Lavender essential oil shampoo

Ingredients:

- Castile soap – ½ cup
- Peppermint essential oil – 10 drops
- Tea tree oil – 10 drops
- Rosemary oil – 10 drops
- Distilled water – ½ cup

Method:

- Pour the castile soap into the bottle that you will use to hold the shampoo.
- Add in the oils along with the distilled water and give the bottle a good shake.
- The shampoo is mild enough to be used every other day.

Note: You can buy the castile soap online on websites such as Amazon or at any good pharmacy.

Hair conditioner

Ingredients:

- Cider vinegar – ½ cup
- Mint essential oil – 10 drops
- Milk powder – 2 tablespoons

Method:

- Mix all the ingredients in a bowl and transfer to a flip-top bottle.
- Use the conditioner after washing hair with the lavender shampoo and rinse off after 2 minutes.

Anti-Aging Serum

Ingredients:

- Carrot seed oil – 10 drops
- Geranium oil – 10 drops
- Sandalwood oil – 10 drops
- Rosemary oil – 10 drops
- Coconut oil – ½ cup
- Lemon oil – 10 drops
- Apricot oil – 10 drops

Method:

- Add all ingredients into a jar and give it a good shake.
- Apply 2-3 drops daily on face and neck.
- With time, the serum will help in reversing signs of aging and render a youthful glow.

Nail scrub and moisturizer

Ingredients:

- Granulated salt – 1/2 cup
- Fuller's Earth – 1 cup
- Lanolin oil – 2 tablespoons
- Petroleum jelly – 2 tablespoons
- Essential oil (rose, lavender, ginger, peppermint, geranium, cypress) – 10 drops

Method:

- Mix all ingredients in a plastic bowl and transfer to a plastic jar.
- The nail scrub can be used as a cuticle softener as well.

Homemade Hand Sanitizer

Hand sanitizers can be used in place of hand washes especially when outdoors.

Ingredients:

- Rose oil – 10 drops
- Tea tree oil – 40 drops
- 100% proof vodka – 1 tablespoon
- Vitamin E oil – ¼ teaspoon

Method:

- Mix everything in a glass bowl and transfer into a small plastic flip top bottle.
- Use coin-sized amount.

Calming and Soothing Foot Concoction

Ingredients:

- Lemon essential oil – 10 drops
- Lavender essential oil – 10 drops
- Tea tree oil – 10 drops

Method:

- Mix all the ingredients in a plastic bottle and shake thoroughly.
- A little mixture can be added to pedicure water or the mixture can be applied to feet before retiring to bed.
- Adding a little Shea butter will help it develop a creamy consistency and make for an easier application.

The concoction will keep infections at bay thanks to the tea tree oil and will also help in keeping feet moisturized.

Minty Soothing Foot Cream

Ingredients:-

- Olive oil - 3 tablespoons
- Emulsifying wax - 2 tablespoons
- Shea butter - 2 tablespoons
- Water - 3/4 cup
- Citric acid - 1 teaspoon
- Peppermint oil - 25 drops
- Tea tree oil - 15 drops

Method:-

- Place a large enough saucepan filled with water over high heat, and bring to a boil. Reduce heat to medium-low and let the water simmer. Place a heat resistant glass bowl on top form a double boiler. Add the water, wax and citric acid. Stir occasionally, until the wax melts. Once the wax mixture is melted and well combined, remove from heat.
- In another small bowl, combine peppermint oil, tea tree oil, olive oil, Shea butter, and whisk for about 60 seconds until well blended.
- Once the wax mixture cools down, add essential oil mixture to it. Whisk to combine well.

- Transfer this mixture to an air-tight container, and use it as a foot cream for relaxation.

Bath Bombs

Bath bombs are small cosmetic toiletries that you can add into your tub or bath water to enhance its therapeutic value.

Ingredients:

- Baking soda – 2 cups
- Citric acid crystals – 1 cup
- Corn flour – 1 cup
- Olive oil – ½ cup
- Essential oils (lavender, rose, sandal, eucalyptus, orange, strawberry, lemon) – 20 drops
- Molds of different shapes
- Witch hazel (optional)

Method:

- Mix all the ingredients in a glass or ceramic bowl (avoid plastic), and stir with a wooden spatula.
- Add in 1-2 teaspoons of witch hazel to help hold it together. However, the mixture should be wet enough to combine together easily.
- Use muffin cup or any silicone mold of your choice and fill each one with the mixture, packing it in tightly.

- Allow it to rest for 12 to 24 hours before slowly removing each from their mold and transferring them into a glass jar.

Add a bomb into your bath water and wait for it to completely dissolve. It will fizzle as it dissolves owing to the citric acid crystals dissolving and reacting with the baking soda.

Perfume

Ingredients:

- Olive oil – ¼ cup
- Essential oils – orange, vanilla, rose – 30 drops each
- 100% proof vodka – ½ cup

Method:

- Mix everything in a glass bowl and transfer into a glass bottle or an emptied and thoroughly cleaned scent bottle.
- The combination of top, base, and middle ingredients will depend on individual preferences.
- Allow the perfume to mature by placing it in a dark room for a couple of days.

Note: naturally, you can mix and match different essential oils to obtain a different scent.

Skin Lotions and Creams

Dry Skin Cream

Ingredients:

- Water – ¼ cup
- Sesame oil – ¼ cup
- Vitamin E oil - 2 ½ teaspoons
- Beeswax (grated) - 2 tablespoons
- Grapefruit essential oil - 3 drops

Method:

- In a bowl, combine bees wax with vitamin E oil, sesame seeds, and mix well.
- Transfer this bowl to a large pan filled with water, and heat it for 20 minutes until the wax melts.
- Now heat the grapefruit oil and water on slow heat for 10-12 minutes. Combine both the mixtures. Once cooled down, store in air-tight containers.

Sesame oil face cream

Ingredients:-

- Sesame oil - 2 tablespoons
- Apricot essential oil - 2 teaspoons
- Vitamin E oil - 2 teaspoons
- Clove essential oil 2 teaspoons
- Cocoa butter – 3.5 oz.

Method:-

- Take a bowl and combine sesame oil, apricot oil, Vitamin E oil, clove oil, and cocoa butter, and mix well using a beater or just stir for about 5-6 minutes using a spatula.
- Put some water in a big pot, and let it heat up for about 5 minutes. Place the bowl containing cocoa butter and oils inside the pot.
- Let this mixture heat for another few minutes until the cocoa butter completely melts. Once the mixture cools, store it in a plastic air-tight container, and use it on your face every night before sleeping.

Green Tea face cream

Ingredients:

- Aloe vera juice – 3 ½ tablespoons
- Hazel nut oil - 4 tablespoons
- Lemon oil - 2 tablespoons
- Emulsifying wax - 2 tablespoons
- Vitamin E - 1 teaspoon
- Citric acid - 1 teaspoon
- Green tea, infused strong – 6 tablespoons

Method:

- Combine wax and all the oils mentioned in the ingredients in a bowl. Heat this bowl over a pot full of water until the wax dissolves.
- Brew the green tea in some water. Now add the oil mixture and citric acid to the green tea. Mix well. Store it in a jar in the refrigerator. Ensure that you are not allergic to Aloe Vera by doing a patch test on your wrist.

Moisturizing lotion

Ingredients:

- Baby lotion – 7 oz.
- coconut oil – ⅓ cup
- vitamin E oil - 3 tablespoons
- Pine essential oil - 1 teaspoon

Method:-

- In a bowl, blend coconut oil, vitamin E oil, pine oil, and baby lotion using a beater or stir for about 7-8minutes using a spoon. Using a hand blender too can be a good alternative as we want all the ingredients to be mixed together without any lumps.
- Fill this mixture in a plastic container, and store in your refrigerator. The pine oil included in this recipe will keep away all the bacteria.

Body Lotion

Ingredients:

- Jojoba oil – ½ cup
- Coconut oil – ½ cup
- Shea butter – ¼ cup
- Cranberry essential oil – 20-25 drops

Method:

- Place all the ingredients on a double boiler, and melt until it reaches a creamy consistency
- Remove from heat and add in the essential oils.
- Give everything a good mix and transfer into a jar.
- The body lotion will keep your skin hydrated for at least 6 hours.

CONCLUSION

I want to thank you for downloading this Book, and for the time you invested with us. We have discussed everything that you need to know about aromatherapy and essential oils in this eBook.

We hope that after learning the beauty benefits of these natural essential oils, you will now incorporate them in your daily beauty regime and reap the amazing benefits that these oils bring with them.

Rather than opting for chemically laced products and treatments, it is best that you rely on Mother Nature's basket for some amazing treatments that will add to your beauty.

In this eBook, we have explained how you can make these essential oils at home and also shared some recipes that will help you make different skin care products from the comforts of your home.

Thanks once again for your time, and we hope you enjoyed reading the book. Hopefully you will try out some of these recipes to make some amazing body baths, body butters, creams, and other beauty essentials

MORE BOOKS FROM JOSEPHINE SIMON

Learn to make your own All-Natural Bath Bombs and Bubble Baths at Home today! It's fun and easy!

Bath bombs and bubble bath make bath time so much more fun and enjoyable for adults and kids alike. The best part is that you can make your own at home. It's that easy. Relax in a luxurious hot bath of bubble and fizzies, rejuvenating and pampering your body, and awakening all your sense.

Just click on the book cover to check it out.

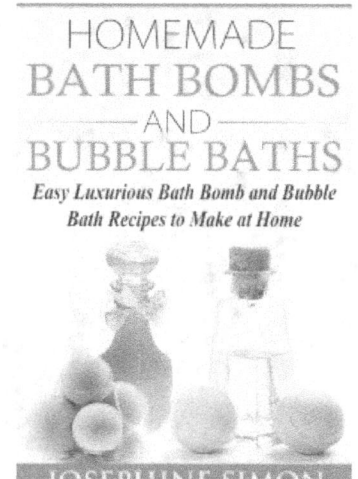

Make your own all-natural beauty products at home. It's easier than you think!

Get ready to pamper yourself and get radiant and youthful skin. It's easier than you think! Learn to prepare your own organic beauty products like body lotions, creams, moisturizers, body scrubs, body butter and more with all-natural ingredients that are hiding in your own kitchen!

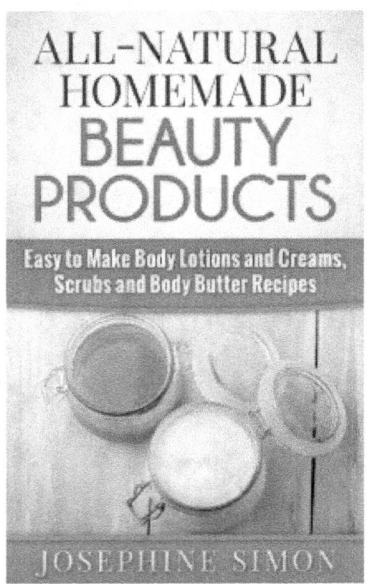